MW01593533

EMMA HEMING WILLIS PERFORMATIVE BOOK:

CARING FOR BRUCE WILLIS, THE UNEXPECTED JOURNEY - A PROSOPOGRAPHY

KINGSLEY PENS

Table of Contents for Emma Heming Willis Performative Book: Caring for Bruce Willis, THE UNEXPECTED JOURNEY – A Prosopography

Introduction

Love in the Spotlight: When Caregiving Becomes the Story

Chapter One

From Runways to Real Life: Emma's Evolution into a Reluctant Advocate

Chapter Two

The Diagnosis That Changed Everything: Facing Frontotemporal Dementia Together

Chapter Three

Public Grace, Private Pain: Navigating the Media and the Moments Between

Chapter Four

Redefining Strength: Motherhood, Marriage, and Mental Health in the Caregiver Role

Chapter Five

The Village Behind the Care: Family, Friends, and the Unseen Hands of Support

Chapter Six

Voicing the Journey: Using Platforms for Awareness, Action, and Advocacy

Chapter Seven

Hope in the Everyday: Finding Beauty, Humor, and Humanity in the Hardest Times

Conclusion

Still With Love: The Ongoing Story of Compassion, Connection, and Courage

Introduction
Love in the Spotlight: When Caregiving Becomes the Story

She never asked for the spotlight to shine in this way. Emma Heming Willis, once known for her striking presence on fashion runways and red carpets, found herself facing a far more intimate and consuming stage. Not the glossy covers of magazines or glamorous galas, but a quiet, often isolating space where love meets responsibility, where marriage becomes a sanctuary, and where caregiving becomes an act of daily courage. When Bruce Willis, the beloved actor known for his iconic roles and larger-than-life screen persona, was diagnosed with frontotemporal dementia, the world gasped. But behind that global gasp was a woman holding her family together, reimagining what it means to be both a wife and a caregiver under public scrutiny.

This is not a story about tragedy. It is a story about unexpected strength, quiet advocacy, and the power of love when everything changes. It is about Emma—mother, wife, protector, and reluctant spokesperson—who stepped into a role she did not choose, but embraced with fierce grace. Her journey, marked by vulnerability and resilience, reflects a broader truth about countless caregivers who walk through similar storms, mostly invisible to the world. Emma's visibility gave those invisible stories a name, a face, and a beating heart.

When we talk about celebrity, we often focus on curated perfection. We see the posed family photos, the carefully worded captions, the manicured lives that seem untouched by the wear and tear of everyday struggle. Emma shattered that illusion—not with bitterness, but with honesty. She chose to share pieces of her journey not for sympathy, but to spread awareness, build community, and humanize the caregiving experience that millions endure in silence. Her vulnerability invited others to breathe, to speak, and to stop pretending.

From the moment Bruce's diagnosis was shared with the world, Emma became more than just a celebrity spouse. She became a witness to the slow fade of a vibrant man, a protector of her children's peace, and a spokesperson for a disease that still lives in the margins of medical and public understanding. Yet, she did not come bearing medical expertise or professional credentials. She came with love—raw, real, unwavering— and a willingness to tell the truth about what caregiving actually looks like behind the curtains.

What makes Emma's journey especially compelling is not just the magnitude of who Bruce Willis is in American culture, but the grace with which she redefined her public identity. She was never trying to steal the narrative. She was merely trying to survive it. In the process, she invited others into the sacred, often unseen work of caregiving. She allowed the world to see that being a caregiver is not about martyrdom. It is about devotion. It is about waking up each day and choosing to love through the fog, through the frustrations, through the fear.

Emma's story echoes the collective experience of many women who become caregivers to their partners. Studies show that women make up the majority of unpaid caregivers in the United States. These women often carry the emotional, physical, and logistical load of care, all while trying to maintain some sense of self.

Emma's willingness to say out loud, "This is hard, and I am not okay every day," became a radical act in a culture that often silences women's pain beneath a polished smile. Her transparency created space for others to admit their own weariness without shame.

Caregiving, especially for someone with dementia, is a layered and emotionally complex role. It means grieving someone while they are still here. It means adjusting to a new version of your loved one, even as you cling to the fragments of who they used to be. It means becoming fluent in patience, in redirecting emotion, in managing unpredictability. Emma never pretended to have all the answers. Instead, she offered presence. She offered honesty. She offered her own story as a bridge for others to walk across.

The love between Emma and Bruce was never meant to be examined under a microscope. But once it became part of the public conversation, Emma made a deliberate choice. She chose to use her voice not just to protect Bruce, but to shine a light on an often overlooked part of the healthcare experience. She partnered with organizations, shared educational resources, and spoke about self-care with refreshing candor. She acknowledged the burnout, the isolation, the guilt, and the longing that caregivers carry. She gave language to the emotional terrain that many are too exhausted to map.

But this introduction is not just a tribute to Emma's strength. It is also a reflection on what it means to love someone through decline, to show up when everything familiar begins to shift. It asks what it means to be a partner when your partner slowly slips into a different version of themselves. It examines the way public identity and private pain intersect, and how one woman found a way to hold both with grace.

Emma's journey also challenges societal narratives around womanhood, marriage, and resilience. Too often, the caregiver is expected to be endlessly strong, endlessly patient, endlessly invisible. But Emma disrupted that expectation. She showed that strength can cry. That patience can take breaks. That invisibility can be replaced with advocacy. She helped redefine what it means to be a wife—not just as a romantic partner, but as a warrior in the trenches of illness, loss, and love.

This story also brings to the forefront the reality of frontotemporal dementia—a disease that does not get the same attention as Alzheimer's but is just as devastating. It strikes younger, progresses differently, and often affects behavior and personality before memory. The challenges are nuanced, the emotional impact unique. Through Emma's public reflections, more people became aware, more families felt less alone, and more attention was given to a disease that had lived in the shadows for too long.

In the world of celebrity, many choose silence when life becomes difficult. Emma chose connection. She used her platform to speak to caregivers, to reach into the hearts of those who knew the weight of her words. She did not speak as a savior, but as someone learning in real time how to navigate loss while holding on to love. Her courage lies not in having overcome, but in being willing to keep showing up every day.

Emma's approach also redefines beauty and success. Once celebrated for her appearance, she became a different kind of icon—a woman who lives with integrity, who speaks with empathy, and who allows her humanity to lead. She reminds us that caregiving is not the end of one's identity but the evolution of it. That we are allowed to be both grieving and grateful. That we can be strong and soft at the same time.

In every image shared, every interview given, and every quiet moment described, Emma reflects a truth that many know but rarely see validated in public life—that caregiving is both a privilege and a burden, that it stretches the soul and reorders priorities, and that love is not always glamorous but is always worth it. Her journey is an invitation to reimagine what devotion looks like, especially when it is tested by illness and illuminated by vulnerability.

This book will explore Emma Heming Willis's unexpected journey through seven transformative chapters, each uncovering a layer of her life as caregiver, wife, mother, and advocate. It will highlight her evolution from model to matriarch, from silent supporter to outspoken advocate. It will trace the impact of Bruce's illness on their marriage, their family, and their public life. It will give voice to the emotional complexity of caregiving and celebrate the quiet victories that come from choosing love again and again in the face of the unknown.

Emma's story is not just about Bruce's illness. It is about how love endures. How identity shifts. How women rise. How families adapt. How truth heals. In the pages ahead, readers will see a portrait not just of Emma Heming Willis, but of every woman who has ever stood in the fire for someone they love and came out bearing light. Through her example, we learn that caregiving, especially in the spotlight, is not about losing yourself—it is about finding a deeper, truer version of who you are.

And in this unexpected journey, that is the most powerful transformation of all.

Chapter One
From Runways to Real Life: Emma's Evolution into a Reluctant Advocate

Long before she became the face of caregiving courage, Emma Heming Willis was known as the graceful beauty who commanded catwalks and magazine covers with poise and polish. Her early life was filled with photo shoots, modeling contracts, and the kind of glamor that often defines success in the public eye. She walked for top designers and became a recognizable figure in the global fashion scene. Her life appeared meticulously curated, a portrait of elegance and ambition. Yet nothing in those years of cameras and couture could have prepared her for the real-life stage she would one day occupy—the deeply human, unfiltered, and relentless world of caregiving.

Emma's transformation from model to matriarch did not happen overnight. It unfolded through subtle shifts and seismic life changes. It began, as many love stories do, with connection. When she met Bruce Willis, the chemistry was undeniable. Their courtship was not defined by flashy headlines or staged appearances, but by a quiet and sincere bond that transcended fame. Bruce, long revered as a Hollywood legend, found in Emma a grounding force, someone who was both graceful and real, someone who did not need the spotlight but who carried light within her.

Marriage brought Emma into a different kind of public visibility. Suddenly she was no longer just Emma Heming, the model, but Emma Heming Willis, the wife of an American icon. With that new name came a new role—one that required balance, discretion, and resilience. She stepped into blended family life with openness, embracing Bruce's daughters from his previous marriage and later welcoming two daughters of their own. Her world expanded to include school runs, family holidays, birthday parties, and the beautifully ordinary moments that make life meaningful. The glitz was still there, but it was softened by the grounding presence of home.

Emma's life, however, took a dramatic turn when Bruce began to show signs that something was not quite right. Subtle changes in behavior, communication, and memory became impossible to ignore. What began as small concerns gradually grew into larger questions. As his condition progressed, Emma was forced to confront a new reality—one that would test every fiber of her emotional strength. The man she loved was changing in front of her eyes, and there was no script, no red carpet, and no easy answers.

The diagnosis of frontotemporal dementia (FTD) was both a blow and a strange kind of relief. It gave a name to the confusion and a shape to the fear. But it also marked the beginning of Emma's next chapter—a chapter she never asked for but would come to embody with breathtaking resilience. Overnight, she became not just a wife and mother, but a full-time caregiver. Her days shifted from modeling projects to managing medical appointments, emotional breakdowns, and the slow unraveling of a partner's identity. She entered a world where beauty was measured not by appearance but by endurance, by the ability to show up, stay present, and love through the loss.

It would have been easy, even understandable, for Emma to retreat. Many in her position might have chosen privacy, disappearing from public view to grieve and cope in silence. But Emma did something quietly revolutionary. She allowed herself to be seen. Not as the picture-perfect spouse, but as a woman learning how to navigate heartbreak in real time. Her Instagram posts changed tone. Her interviews became more personal. She began speaking not just about Bruce, but about the millions of caregivers who walk similar paths, hidden in plain sight.

What made Emma's evolution so compelling was her refusal to paint over the pain. She did not perform strength. She lived it. And in doing so, she gave others permission to be honest about their own caregiving experiences. She shared her struggles with setting boundaries, with managing her own mental health, with making time for herself in the midst of unending responsibility. She talked about guilt, about exhaustion, and about the need to ask for help. These admissions were not signs of weakness. They were acts of advocacy.

Through her vulnerability, Emma became a reluctant but powerful voice for those who rarely get to speak. She began partnering with organizations focused on brain health and caregiving. She shared resources, amplified the stories of other families affected by dementia, and used her platform to shine a light on the invisible labor carried out every day by spouses, children, and loved ones across the world. What began as a personal journey became a public mission.

Emma never sought this role. She did not set out to become an advocate. But like so many women before her, she rose to meet the moment. Not because she was unafraid, but because she loved too deeply to look away. Her journey shows us that advocacy does not always start in protest or on a podium. Sometimes it starts in the kitchen, holding a cup of coffee at dawn, wondering how you will get through another day. Sometimes it begins with a whisper, a confession, a plea for understanding. And sometimes it grows from the simple act of choosing to love someone even as they forget pieces of who they were.

Her advocacy also challenged the cultural expectations placed on women in caregiving roles. Too often, society expects women to bear suffering silently, to be grateful for the opportunity to care, even as they lose themselves in the process. Emma disrupted that narrative. She insisted that caregivers are not saints, but humans. That they need support, community, rest, and recognition. She spoke about the importance of therapy, of self-compassion, and of acknowledging grief even while a loved one is still alive. She reframed caregiving not as a burden to be hidden, but as a complex act of love that deserves to be seen.

In sharing her story, Emma helped normalize the emotional rollercoaster of loving someone through cognitive decline. She did not sugarcoat the hard days. She admitted to crying, to being overwhelmed, to feeling lost.

But she also spoke about the moments of connection that still surfaced, the flickers of humor and tenderness that made it all worthwhile. These glimpses of joy amidst sorrow gave hope to others. They reminded caregivers that it is okay to feel everything at once—grief, love, fatigue, hope—and that no one has to do this alone.

Her daughters became part of the story too. Emma opened up about how she navigates the challenge of raising young girls while also caring for their father. She spoke about the importance of honesty, of letting her children see that sadness is not something to hide, but something to move through together. In doing so, she modeled a kind of emotional intelligence that will shape their understanding of love, family, and strength for the rest of their lives.

Emma's evolution into advocacy was not marked by a singular moment. It unfolded quietly, in the small choices she made every day. The choice to speak. The choice to show up. The choice to give love even when it hurt. And it is this quiet power that makes her story resonate so deeply. She is not a hero in the traditional sense. She is something braver—a woman who stepped into an unwelcome storm and found a way to carry others through it with her.

The transition from runways to real life is not just a metaphor. It is a truth that defines Emma's journey. She walked away from a world that celebrated surface beauty and entered one where beauty is defined by patience, presence, and perseverance. She redefined what it means to be seen—not just in photographs, but in pain, in growth, and in service to someone you love. She showed that caregiving is not the end of a woman's identity, but the beginning of a deeper understanding of who she is.

Emma Heming Willis never asked for this role. But she stepped into it with clarity, courage, and compassion. Her evolution reminds us that real life does not care for scripts or perfect lighting. It unfolds in unpredictable ways. It asks us to grow. To stretch. To surrender and to rise. And in Emma's case, it reveals a woman who continues to redefine what it means to love with everything you have, even when everything is changing.

Her story is not about losing a husband to illness. It is about holding on to love through transformation. It is about showing up for the people you care about, even when the path is unclear. It is about using your voice, not because you want attention, but because you know someone else needs to hear that they are not alone.

Emma's journey from the runway to the rawness of caregiving is not just a personal evolution. It is a collective mirror. It reflects what many women go through behind closed doors. It brings the private into the public and dares to say, "This matters." Through her strength and her softness, she invites all of us to think differently about what it means to care, to advocate, and to love without conditions. And in doing so, she has become not just a reluctant advocate, but a luminous one.

Chapter Two

The Diagnosis That Changed Everything: Facing Frontotemporal Dementia Together

There is a moment in every life where the world tilts. One phone call, one doctor's visit, one sentence can fracture what once felt familiar and safe. For Emma Heming Willis, that moment arrived wrapped in uncertainty, fear, and heartbreak. The man she loved, Bruce Willis, the father of her children, the charismatic force known to millions, was diagnosed with frontotemporal dementia. From that moment on, life was no longer about red carpets or rehearsed lines. It became about navigating a reality where clarity faded, words slipped away, and time began to stretch and collapse in unpredictable ways.

At first, the signs were subtle. There were pauses in conversations that felt out of place. Moments of confusion that did not match Bruce's usual sharpness. He might forget a word mid-sentence or repeat himself in a way that made Emma's heart pause. These changes arrived quietly, cloaked in normalcy, often explained away by stress, age, or fatigue. But Emma, like so many partners tuned into their loved one's rhythms, knew something was wrong.

The most terrifying part of those early days was not knowing what they were facing. Emma watched the man who had once delivered punchlines and action lines with effortless charisma begin to fumble over simple exchanges. There were good days and not-so-good days, which made it even harder to accept that something irreversible was unfolding. When the doctors began to run tests, when the appointments became routine, when specialists began mentioning neurological evaluations, the reality began to settle in. But it was the official diagnosis—frontotemporal dementia—that changed everything.

Frontotemporal dementia, or FTD, is a cruel thief. Unlike Alzheimer's, which is more commonly recognized and begins with memory loss, FTD targets the front and temporal lobes of the brain. These are the parts responsible for personality, behavior, and language. It is the kind of condition that alters how a person interacts with the world, how they speak, and how they understand what others are saying. It does not just affect memory. It reshapes identity. And it arrives early, often affecting people in their forties, fifties, or sixties—those very years when life is supposed to be in full bloom.

For Emma, the diagnosis was both devastating and clarifying. It confirmed what her heart already knew, but it also forced her into a reality she had no roadmap for. The man she married would not fade in the ways most people imagine. He would remain physically strong, his smile still radiant, but his words and behaviors would change. Slowly, subtly, then more significantly. She would have to become fluent in a new language of care. A new way of loving. A new version of presence.

One of the most agonizing parts of the diagnosis was explaining it to their daughters. How do you tell young children that their father is changing and that those changes are permanent? Emma chose honesty wrapped in compassion. She spoke to them not with fear but with gentleness. She let them ask questions. She encouraged them to express confusion, frustration, and sadness. She did not pretend to have all the answers, but she gave them what every child deserves—truth, stability, and love.

Emma also had to learn to grieve someone who was still here. That is the particular cruelty of FTD. The person you love sits beside you, holds your hand, smiles at you, but pieces of them begin to drift. There are moments when they are fully themselves—laughing at a joke, enjoying music, recalling a memory—and then moments when the fog moves in and you are reminded that the man you love is changing in ways neither of you can control. It is a grief that is ongoing, layered, and unpredictable.

Despite the pain, Emma made a decision early on: they would face this together. She would not retreat into despair, nor would she allow their home to become defined solely by illness. Instead, she committed to building a life that could hold both joy and sorrow, clarity and confusion. She chose to honor the man Bruce had been while embracing the man he was becoming. In doing so, she demonstrated a kind of love that goes beyond romance—a love built on devotion, adaptability, and faith.

One of the first challenges Emma encountered was learning about the medical and emotional complexities of FTD. It is a condition that lacks public understanding and often gets misdiagnosed. Many families struggle for years before receiving a correct diagnosis. Emma immersed herself in the research. She sought out specialists, read everything she could, and began building a care team that understood not just Bruce's medical needs, but his humanity. She became his advocate, his voice in appointments, and his comfort in moments of uncertainty.

And then there was the public. Bruce Willis was not just her husband. He was a beloved figure around the world. The world had watched him leap from explosions, deliver iconic one-liners, and light up the screen for decades. Now, the same world would watch him disappear in a different way. Emma understood that the diagnosis would not stay private forever. So when the time came to share the news publicly, she chose transparency. She released a statement that was honest, dignified, and filled with love. She acknowledged the pain, highlighted the importance of awareness, and asked for grace.

That decision opened a new chapter. Suddenly, Emma was not just a wife and caregiver. She was the face of a condition that many had never heard of. Messages poured in from families around the world—people who were walking similar paths, who felt seen by her words, who thanked her for speaking out. Emma realized that by telling her story, she could help others feel less alone. She could use her visibility to draw attention to a disease that had remained in the shadows for too long.

But advocacy came with a cost. Every time she spoke about Bruce's condition, it meant reliving the pain. It meant inviting strangers into the most vulnerable parts of her life. Still, Emma kept showing up. Not because it was easy, but because she believed in the power of truth. She believed in community. She believed that awareness could lead to funding, to research, to hope for future families. And through it all, she remained fiercely protective of Bruce's dignity. She never shared more than was necessary. She never sensationalized his condition. She offered glimpses, not for drama, but for connection.

Life after the diagnosis became a study in adaptation. Emma learned to slow down. She learned to celebrate small victories—days when Bruce was lucid, meals shared without confusion, quiet moments of eye contact. She created routines that brought stability. Music, nature, and family rituals became anchors. She taught their daughters that love does not fade with illness. It evolves. It deepens. It stretches to hold what words can no longer express.

There were hard days too—days when Bruce grew agitated, when communication broke down, when Emma felt utterly depleted. There were nights when the weight of it all seemed unbearable. But even in those moments, she never stopped choosing love. She cried when she needed to. She reached out for support. She practiced grace with herself. And slowly, she began to understand that facing this diagnosis was not about fixing what was broken. It was about being present in what remained.

Emma's experience also revealed the cracks in the system—the lack of resources for families facing FTD, the emotional toll on caregivers, and the invisibility of the labor involved. She used her voice to advocate for change. She spoke about the need for better access to care, for caregiver support, and for a culture that values emotional labor. Her honesty sparked conversations across the caregiving and medical communities, elevating voices that had long gone unheard.

At the heart of Emma's journey was a truth many caregivers come to know: that love is not always a feeling. Sometimes, it is a decision. A discipline. A quiet vow to stay when things are no longer easy. Bruce's diagnosis did not end their love story. It transformed it. It made it messier, more sacred, and more real. Emma learned to love him not for what he remembered, but for who he was in the moment. She discovered that even in silence, connection remains. Even in decline, dignity endures.

Facing frontotemporal dementia together became an act of resistance. Against despair. Against invisibility. Against the erasure of those affected. It became a way to reclaim agency in the face of uncertainty. And through Emma's lens, we see that this journey—though filled with pain—is also filled with meaning. That within the hardest days live the most tender moments. That caregiving, when rooted in love, becomes a form of quiet revolution.

As Emma continued to walk this road, she did not pretend to have all the answers. But she remained committed to walking it with intention, with integrity, and with open hands. Her story reminds us that a diagnosis does not define a life. It reshapes it. It invites us to listen more closely, to hold each other more tightly, and to speak even when the words are hard to find.

In the face of one of life's most profound challenges, Emma Heming Willis became something more than a wife or caregiver. She became a mirror for all who are navigating similar terrain. A reminder that we are not alone. That our stories matter. And that even when the world tilts, love can still be the thing that holds everything together.

Chapter Three

Public Grace, Private Pain: Navigating the Media and the Moments Between

There is a delicate tension that exists when a person lives at the intersection of public admiration and private anguish. For Emma Heming Willis, that tension became the soundtrack of her life. The world knew her as Bruce Willis's wife, a poised figure of strength, beauty, and grace. Cameras caught her in polished attire, gently holding Bruce's hand, offering soft smiles and words of encouragement during public appearances. To outsiders, she exuded serenity. But behind those smiles lived a reality marked by exhaustion, heartbreak, and the countless quiet moments where she cried in solitude.

From the moment Bruce's health began to change, the public eye never strayed far. He was, after all, not just any actor. Bruce Willis was an icon—an emblem of cinematic masculinity, the star of blockbusters, and a household name across generations. When whispers of his cognitive decline first circulated in the media, speculation quickly swelled. There were photos of him looking distant, stories wondering about his absence from the screen, and rumors that careened across tabloids without fact or compassion. Emma watched as her husband's legacy was dissected by strangers who had no understanding of what he was truly facing.

Navigating the media became a balancing act. Emma had to decide how much of their reality to share and how much to keep sacred. She knew that silence could lead to dangerous speculation, yet transparency could invite intrusion. With intentionality and courage, she stepped forward to tell the truth—but on her terms. The family's public statement about Bruce's diagnosis was a model of dignity. It honored his journey, respected his humanity, and asked for compassion. But what the world did not see was the tremble in her voice as she approved the wording, the way her fingers lingered on the send button, or how she stayed awake that night, bracing for the wave of responses.

The response was immediate. News outlets ran the story across front pages and news tickers. Celebrities offered support, fans shared memories, and caregivers across the globe reached out with empathy. Yet even amidst that wave of compassion, Emma felt exposed. Every post she made, every step outside her home, became part of a story larger than she had chosen. She was not just managing a household in crisis. She was managing a narrative—a global perception of who they were and how they were coping.

But Emma refused to let the media script her story. Instead, she became a careful curator of truth. Through social media, she offered glimpses of their life—not curated for perfection, but chosen with purpose. She shared photos of Bruce playing with their daughters, moments of stillness in the garden, videos filled with laughter and light. These images weren't meant to mask the pain. They were a declaration: joy still lives here. Life, though altered, is still full of connection, presence, and love.

Behind the camera, however, the picture was more complicated. Emma bore the weight of constant worry. She juggled doctor appointments, therapy sessions, and the emotional labor of supporting her children while trying to process her own grief. Her days were filled with routine—ensuring Bruce had his medication, preparing meals, creating environments that felt calm and safe. And all the while, the outside world continued to gaze in, commenting, praising, sometimes even judging.

Public grace required private strength. Emma had to master the art of appearing calm when inside she was unraveling. There were days she stood in front of a mirror, forcing a smile because she knew the media would capture her face. There were mornings when the grief sat so heavily on her chest that she could barely breathe, but she still made it through school drop-offs and interviews. She learned how to be composed even as her life was coming undone in ways the world could not see.

The moments between—the ones without cameras, without statements, without filters—were the most sacred and the most painful. These were the quiet spaces where the true cost of caregiving lived. The evenings when Bruce would forget something deeply familiar, and Emma would step into the role of calm navigator. The nights when he would ask a question she had already answered five times, and she would offer the sixth response with the same loving tone. The days when he did not seem to recognize a friend's face, or when a song no longer stirred memory. Each of these instances etched a deeper layer of heartbreak into Emma's soul.

But they also revealed her resilience. In these private moments, Emma discovered a strength that could not be captured in headlines. She became fluent in the language of patience. She learned to find comfort in the smallest victories—a shared smile, a completed sentence, a peaceful afternoon. She adjusted her expectations and clung to the present, knowing that each day with Bruce as he was in that moment was a gift.

She also became intimately familiar with the duality of emotions. There were days filled with both laughter and tears, joy and sorrow. One moment Bruce might be dancing in the kitchen with their daughters, and the next he might struggle to remember the steps. Emma learned to ride the emotional waves without letting them consume her. She cried when she needed to. She screamed into pillows. She journaled her fears. She prayed. And in the quietest of hours, when everyone else was asleep, she sat with her feelings and gave herself permission to grieve what was lost and to cherish what remained.

Navigating the media spotlight also meant protecting Bruce's legacy. Emma was determined that his public image would reflect dignity, not pity. She pushed back against narratives that framed him as a tragedy. Instead, she championed the truth that Bruce was still here, still loving, still laughing, still showing up for life in his own way. This required fierce intentionality. Every photo she shared, every word she spoke, carried the weight of that mission.

But advocacy also opened doors. Through her visibility, Emma began collaborating with organizations focused on frontotemporal dementia. She joined conversations that previously felt too medical, too removed from everyday families. She brought heart and story to clinical conversations. She helped raise awareness for a condition that desperately needed public attention. Her voice became a bridge between science and humanity, between policy and lived experience.

Still, advocacy was never her end goal. Her primary calling was care—care for Bruce, care for her children, and care for herself. This last piece, the care of self, was the hardest to learn. For a long time, Emma believed that strength meant sacrifice, that to be a good caregiver, she had to give everything of herself. But eventually, she learned that true resilience requires rest. She began carving out moments just for her—a morning walk, a therapy session, a quiet bath. She learned that caring for herself was not selfish. It was necessary.

In these quiet acts of self-compassion, Emma began to reclaim pieces of her own identity. She rediscovered her love of writing, of being in nature, of connecting with friends who knew her beyond her public role. She surrounded herself with a circle of women who held space for her without expectation, who allowed her to be vulnerable, messy, and unfiltered. Through them, she remembered that she was more than a headline. More than a caregiver. She was a woman still becoming.

Emma's journey through public grace and private pain illuminates a broader truth about the human experience. So many people carry silent burdens while the world watches only the polished version. They smile while aching. They show up while unraveling. And yet, within that contradiction lies extraordinary beauty. Because what Emma showed the world—through her choices, her voice, and her unwavering love—is that grace is not the absence of pain. It is the decision to keep showing up with softness, with honesty, and with open arms.

Her story also redefines what it means to be strong. Strength is not about suppressing emotions. It is about holding space for all of them. It is about crying and continuing. About mourning and making breakfast. About sitting in the dark and still finding ways to light a candle. Emma embodies this strength not because she never breaks, but because she always chooses to rebuild.

In the months that followed the public announcement, Emma continued to walk the line between public figure and private warrior. She spoke at events, lent her name to campaigns, and offered her platform to elevate others. But she also guarded her family's peace. She said no when she needed to. She set boundaries. She protected Bruce's right to be more than a patient. And through it all, she never stopped loving him—not as the actor the world revered, but as the man she built a life with.

The dance between public and private, between grace and grief, continues every day. And while Emma may never have chosen this journey, she has chosen how to walk it—with intention, with integrity, and with extraordinary love. In her story, we find permission to feel deeply, to struggle openly, and to know that strength and softness can live side by side.

She reminds us that behind every public face is a private story. And within every quiet struggle is a lesson in how to love, how to endure, and how to become something braver than we ever imagined. Through Emma, we see that caregiving is not just a role. It is a calling. A sacred act of love that, when held with grace, can change not only the person you care for— but the world watching you.

Chapter Four

Redefining Strength: Motherhood, Marriage, and Mental Health in the Caregiver Role

Strength, in the traditional sense, has often been portrayed as stoic and silent, an unyielding force that stands tall against the storm. But Emma Heming Willis has come to understand strength in a different light—one rooted not in silence, but in vulnerability, not in perfection, but in persistence. As a wife, mother, and caregiver navigating the profound challenges of frontotemporal dementia within her family, Emma's journey has redefined strength through the lens of tenderness, exhaustion, and the everyday choices to keep showing up.

Motherhood is never simple, even under the most stable circumstances. But raising children while simultaneously tending to the emotional and physical needs of a beloved spouse in cognitive decline demands a unique kind of resilience. For Emma, this meant waking up each day with two equally important responsibilities—protecting her daughters' innocence while preparing them, gently, for the changing reality of their father's presence.

Their daughters, still young and bright-eyed, did not fully understand the transformation occurring within their father. One day Bruce was fully engaged in a game, laughing and telling stories, and the next he seemed distant or confused. Emma became their emotional translator, bridging the gap between what they witnessed and what they could comprehend. She answered their questions with honesty wrapped in comfort. She found ways to explain that Daddy's brain was changing, not because of anything he or they had done, but because life sometimes offers challenges that have no clear answers.

This dual responsibility—caring for a spouse and raising children—required Emma to exist in a constant state of vigilance. She had to be present for her daughters' ballet recitals and school projects while also being present for Bruce's neurologist appointments and medication schedules. She had to be both soft and strong, nurturing and commanding, a mother and a medical assistant. The emotional toll of this balancing act was immense, and there were many days when she felt like she was failing in every direction. Yet her daughters' laughter, their hugs, their innate ability to find joy even in the cracks of their world reminded her that love, more than perfection, was the foundation they needed.

Marriage, too, transformed under the weight of Bruce's illness. The vows Emma once spoke— *for better or for worse, in sickness and in health*—became living, breathing promises. But no one prepares for what it means when "sickness" becomes the center of every conversation, every plan, every future hope.

Emma had to learn how to love Bruce in his new form, to find connection where words had started to falter, and to honor the man he had been while adjusting to the man he was becoming.

There were moments of profound sorrow in this shift. Emma grieved the spontaneous conversations, the witty remarks, the private jokes they once shared. She missed the way he used to surprise her with his confidence, the way he anchored their family with his charismatic presence. And yet, within the grief, she found something deeper—an enduring tenderness. She discovered new ways to express love, through touch, through tone, through shared silence. Marriage no longer relied on dialogue, but on presence. On simply being near, holding hands, listening to music together, or sitting in the stillness of the moment.

Still, the emotional labor of caregiving often pushed Emma to the brink. She found herself emotionally exhausted, physically drained, and spiritually stretched. At first, she tried to push through. She wore a mask of optimism and kept a schedule that left little room for rest. But as the days turned into months, and the responsibility deepened, she began to recognize that unrelenting self-sacrifice was not sustainable. Something had to change.

This awakening led Emma to confront an often overlooked aspect of caregiving: mental health. The silent epidemic among caregivers is the expectation to be everything for everyone while neglecting their own needs. Emma realized that in order to care for Bruce and their daughters, she first had to learn how to care for herself. This did not come easily. Guilt often crept in when she took a moment for herself, a walk alone, a call with a friend, or a quiet morning meditation. But she came to understand that self-care was not selfish—it was survival.

Therapy became a lifeline. Speaking with professionals who could hold her pain without judgment gave Emma space to unravel, to grieve, and to heal. She talked about her fears—of losing Bruce piece by piece, of her children growing up too fast under the weight of adult realities, of losing herself in the process. These sessions became sacred spaces where Emma was not a caregiver, not a public figure, but simply a woman doing her best.

She also began to speak more openly about mental health, both privately and publicly. In doing so, she gave other caregivers permission to be honest about their struggles. Her platform became a place not just for awareness of frontotemporal dementia, but for awareness of the emotional realities that accompany the caregiver role. She broke down stigmas and opened conversations that had long been hidden in shame. And by sharing her story, she invited others to do the same.

Emma's days still follow a rhythm that blends motherhood, marriage, and caregiving. She wakes early, prepares her daughters for school, checks in with Bruce, schedules appointments, manages logistics, and tries to carve out moments for her own wellness. Each task is a thread in the intricate tapestry of her life. Some days, the threads feel tangled and frayed. Other days, they align in surprising harmony. But always, the fabric of her strength remains intact—not because it is unbreakable, but because it is real.

The redefining of strength also involved community. Emma learned that asking for help was not a sign of weakness but of wisdom. She surrounded herself with people who could support her—family members, friends, therapists, educators, and medical professionals. She let others carry parts of the burden, even when it felt uncomfortable to let go. In doing so, she modeled for her daughters what it means to be resilient through interdependence rather than isolation.

This village of support allowed her to keep the home environment steady. Bruce continued to be included in family rituals, celebrated for his presence rather than pitied for his limitations. The girls learned empathy by living it. They saw their mother show up, again and again, even on hard days. They saw that strength could look like tears, that bravery could sound like saying, "I need help," and that love is not diminished by illness—it is revealed more clearly through it.

Emma's journey teaches a profound truth: caregiving is not a detour from life. It is life in its most essential form. It is a practice in presence, in sacrifice, in grace. It strips away the superficial and brings into sharp focus what truly matters. In the quiet hours of the night, when the house is finally still and the world outside is unaware, Emma reflects on all that she carries. It is weighty. But it is also sacred.

The role she never asked for has become a calling. Not because she chose the circumstances, but because she chose how to respond to them—with faithfulness, with openness, and with an evolving understanding of strength. Her life now is not the one she imagined. But it is a life marked by deep love, fierce loyalty, and an inner power that cannot be captured in headlines.

Motherhood, marriage, and mental health—each thread weaves into the portrait of a woman rising. Not out of perfection. Not out of ease. But out of love. Emma has shown that to be a caregiver is to walk a road with no clear end, full of shifting landscapes, and unpredictable turns. But she walks it with eyes wide open, with arms ready to embrace the unknown, and with a heart that, though bruised, beats stronger each day.

In her quiet bravery, we find a redefinition of strength. It is not found in stoicism, but in softness. Not in isolation, but in community. Not in hiding the struggle, but in speaking it out loud. Emma's story is a mirror for every caregiver who has ever doubted their worth, for every mother who has felt stretched too thin, for every wife mourning a slow goodbye. Her life is proof that grace grows in the cracks, and that love, when tested, only deepens.

Through Emma Heming Willis, we see a woman holding it all—the heartbreak, the hope, the exhaustion, the joy. And in her, we recognize a blueprint for what it means to redefine strength not by how little we feel, but by how fully we love.

Chapter Five

The Village Behind the Care: Family, Friends, and the Unseen Hands of Support

Behind every story of strength is a community that often goes unnoticed. In the case of Emma Heming Willis, the face of resilience and compassion in the public eye, that community—her village—is made up of people whose contributions are not always seen or celebrated, but without whom the journey would be unbearable. The caregiving path she walks with Bruce is one woven with profound love and unimaginable weight, but she does not walk it alone. Around her, a circle of family, friends, professionals, and kind-hearted souls have gathered to offer support, wisdom, and quiet acts of grace.

In a society that often glorifies independence, the reality is that no one endures hardship in isolation and survives it intact. Emma learned early in her caregiving journey that asking for help was not a weakness, but a necessity. The demands of supporting a partner with frontotemporal dementia while parenting two young daughters are more than any one person can sustain. To endure, to preserve the quality of life for Bruce and their children, and to protect her own well-being, she had to open her heart and her home to others.

Family, in Emma's case, became both her anchor and her lifeline. Bruce's adult daughters from his previous marriage—Rumer, Scout, and Tallulah—have been not only family but companions on this journey. Their bond with Emma evolved into something deeper than a blended household—it became a united front. There is no roadmap for navigating such a complex family dynamic amid a neurodegenerative illness, but love, communication, and shared purpose forged their path. These women, with their own lives and careers, stepped in with care and reverence for their father, and with tenderness toward Emma and the younger girls.

Their presence in the home created a sense of continuity for Bruce. He saw familiar faces, heard voices that anchored him in memory, and felt the love of daughters who never stopped seeing him for who he truly is. They brought laughter into the home, sat beside him during moments of silence, helped with simple tasks, and relieved Emma of the constant pressure to be everywhere at once. The daughters also became advocates, sharing in the responsibility of educating the public, raising awareness, and maintaining Bruce's dignity in the media spotlight.

But the support did not end there. Emma's own parents, her siblings, and a few deeply trusted friends became the inner circle she leaned on when the days became too long and the emotional weight too heavy. They offered more than just logistical help. They brought companionship, warmth, and the sense that Emma could collapse without fear of judgment. Her mother would cook meals that nourished the family's body and spirit. A sister would take the children for an afternoon so Emma could rest. Friends would stop by simply to sit in silence or hold space for her tears.

There is something sacred about these gestures. The village does not always fix the pain, but it carries some of the weight. The unsung heroes—those who bring groceries, those who remember birthdays, those who text without needing replies—hold up the structure when the foundation threatens to crack. For

Emma, these people are not side characters in her story. They are the scaffolding that holds everything together.

Professional caregivers also entered the picture with grace and dedication. Emma, understanding the complexity of Bruce's diagnosis, knew that professional help was not optional but vital. Nurses, occupational therapists, speech therapists, and home health aides became essential threads in the fabric of care. These professionals came into the home not just with skill, but with compassion. They learned Bruce's patterns, adapted to his rhythms, and treated him with humanity and respect. They offered Emma something rare: peace of mind. Knowing that Bruce was in competent and loving hands allowed her to step back when needed, to be wife and mother again rather than always being nurse and coordinator.

These professionals also brought Emma into a network of knowledge. Through them, she learned how to adjust the environment to support Bruce's needs, how to communicate more effectively, and how to recognize signs of progression without panicking. Their expertise became her confidence, and their guidance became her strength. They were not just caregivers to Bruce. They were mentors to her.

Community support extended beyond the home as well. Teachers at the girls' school provided extra sensitivity and understanding. When a tough morning at home made it hard for the children to focus in class, teachers responded with empathy, not reprimand. Other parents, aware of the family's situation, extended kindness in countless ways—from organizing carpool rides to offering playdates that gave the children a sense of normalcy. These acts, though small on the surface, represented the quiet resilience of a compassionate village.

In a digital age, even strangers became part of Emma's support system. Through social media, messages of encouragement poured in from people who had never met her but felt connected through shared experience. Caregivers from around the world reached out with tips, stories, and solidarity. Their words reminded Emma that she was not alone, and their vulnerability gave her the courage to keep sharing her truth. She built friendships with women across time zones who knew, intimately, the ache and beauty of loving someone with dementia.

Emma found herself both giving and receiving in this global village of care. She was uplifted by others' resilience, and she, in turn, became a beacon for those in earlier stages of the journey. Her willingness to show both the light and the shadows gave others permission to feel, to falter, and to grow. It became clear that caregiving is not just a medical or logistical role. It is a profoundly communal one. It calls on us to love deeper, to lean harder, and to let others in.

Still, allowing the village to help was not always easy. There were moments when Emma struggled with the impulse to do everything herself. She feared being perceived as weak, or worse, as failing. But over time, she learned that true strength does not come from isolation. It comes from trust. From letting others carry parts of the load. From understanding that shared sorrow is lighter, and shared joy is richer.

Emma also faced moments of vulnerability in asking for help from Bruce's close friends.

These were people who had known him before the illness, who had shared film sets and family dinners and inside jokes. Inviting them into the reality of his condition was painful, but it was also healing. Friends like these brought memories into the room—stories of past adventures, photos that sparked recognition, and voices that could still make Bruce smile. They did not come with pity. They came with love, and that love reminded Bruce and Emma both of a life still very much worth living.

Among the unseen hands of support were also those who worked behind the scenes—assistants, housekeepers, coordinators. People whose names may never appear in articles but whose presence ensured that the family could function. Their consistency, their discretion, and their quiet loyalty created an ecosystem where Emma could focus on what mattered most: care, connection, and presence.

Faith also played a role in shaping Emma's village. Prayer groups, spiritual mentors, and sacred rituals brought comfort in ways that transcended words. In times when answers were elusive, faith held her steady. When Emma knelt in silence, she felt surrounded not only by the people in her life but by a divine presence that whispered: you are held. You are not doing this alone.

The power of Emma's village lies in its diversity. Each person offers something different—a hot meal, a shoulder, a joke, a song, a moment of stillness. Together, they form a symphony of support. They are the reason she can rise again and again. They are the quiet force behind every brave choice she makes, the invisible arms catching her when she stumbles.

In a world that often tells women to be everything and to do it alone, Emma's life is a revolutionary testament to the strength of community. Her story reminds us that independence is not the highest form of strength—interdependence is. To let others in, to be honest about the need for help, to surround ourselves with those who see us fully and love us anyway—that is courage.

The caregiving journey is not one path, walked solo. It is a winding road navigated with many hands. Through Emma's story, we see that the village does more than lighten the burden. It enriches the journey. It teaches us about humility, about compassion, and about the beautiful truth that love multiplies when shared.

As Bruce continues to walk his path with dignity and grace, and as Emma continues to guide their family with fierce devotion, it is the village—quiet, steadfast, ever-present—that makes it possible. Behind the scenes, beyond the spotlight, they are the heartbeat of hope. And in their presence, we are reminded that none of us is truly alone. Not in grief. Not in care. Not in love.

Chapter Six
Voicing the Journey: Using Platforms for Awareness, Action, and Advocacy

When Emma Heming Willis first stepped into the public eye, it was through the glamorous world of fashion, beauty, and Hollywood. She was known for her elegance, her composure, and the quiet grace with which she navigated the spotlight. But no photoshoot, red carpet, or magazine spread could have prepared her for the moment when her life demanded a different kind of presence—one that required not poise for the camera, but vulnerability for the world to see.

Emma did not set out to become an advocate. There was no carefully constructed strategy, no media campaign, no grand plan. There was only the raw truth of her husband's diagnosis—frontotemporal dementia—and the life-altering journey it forced her to begin. Suddenly, the woman once admired for her beauty and style found herself confronting a brutal reality, and with it came an unexpected calling: to use her voice not for celebrity, but for something far more sacred.

The decision to go public with Bruce Willis's diagnosis was not one made lightly. It was, in many ways, a moment of reckoning. Emma and the rest of the family knew that Bruce's condition would not remain hidden forever. Rumors had already begun to swirl. People noticed the changes in his public appearances, his absence from film sets, and the subtle shifts in his demeanor. Choosing to share the truth became less about controlling a narrative and more about offering clarity, dignity, and purpose.

By choosing transparency, Emma reclaimed the power of their story. In doing so, she also created space for countless other families walking the same lonely road. Her voice—measured, compassionate, and authentic—cut through the noise of tabloid speculation. She did not sensationalize Bruce's condition, nor did she frame herself as a hero. Instead, she offered something far more powerful: honesty.

In her first public statements, Emma spoke from the heart. She shared how the diagnosis had impacted their family, how the days were filled with both sorrow and love, and how she was learning, moment by moment, how to be a better caregiver, partner, and mother. The public response was overwhelming—not in scandal or pity, but in solidarity. Thousands of messages poured in from people who had been silently carrying similar burdens. Caregivers, spouses, siblings, and children of those with neurodegenerative diseases saw themselves in Emma. Her courage became a mirror reflecting their own.

Recognizing the reach of her platform, Emma began to lean into advocacy more intentionally. She started using her social media not just to update followers, but to educate them. Her posts included practical insights, reflections on caregiving, and resources for those navigating dementia. She uplifted the work of medical professionals, shared articles from neurological research organizations, and directed her audience to trustworthy sources like the Association for Frontotemporal Degeneration (AFTD).

This shift in focus was more than a change in content—it was a transformation of purpose. Emma had once used social media to celebrate fashion and family moments, but now she used it to break down complex ideas into compassionate dialogue. She was still the same woman, but her message had evolved. Now, she was telling the truth of a life that was not curated or filtered, but raw and real.

What made Emma's advocacy so compelling was that it never lost its humanity. She did not posture as an expert or pretend to have all the answers. She often acknowledged her limitations, her fears, and her learning process. She highlighted the emotional toll of caregiving, the mental health challenges that come with watching a loved one decline, and the strength that comes from asking for help. Her vulnerability gave others permission to speak their truth.

Emma also took her advocacy beyond the digital world. She began participating in campaigns and events aimed at increasing awareness of frontotemporal dementia and related conditions. She collaborated with healthcare organizations and researchers, lending her voice to fundraising efforts and awareness drives. When she spoke on panels or gave interviews, she emphasized that early detection, public education, and support networks are critical components of managing these illnesses.

Importantly, Emma always centered the humanity of those affected. She reminded audiences that frontotemporal dementia is not just a diagnosis—it is a lived experience. It affects not only the individual but the entire family system. She spoke of Bruce not as a patient, but as a man still full of dignity, humor, and love. In doing so, she challenged the stigmas that often surround neurological decline. She invited people to see beyond the symptoms and into the heart of the person living through them.

As her advocacy work deepened, Emma began to hear stories from people around the world. Stories of loss and resilience, of heartbreak and healing. People sent her photos of their loved ones, journals of their caregiving days, and thank-you letters for giving their pain a voice. These messages became a part of her purpose. Each one reminded her why speaking up mattered.

She used these stories to amplify the collective experience. In interviews and op-eds, she wove in the words of others, ensuring that her platform was not just about her own journey, but about a shared struggle. She championed policy changes that supported caregivers, including better workplace protections, increased research funding, and improved access to mental health resources. Her voice, once rooted in personal grief, had grown into a public force for change.

And yet, Emma remained grounded. She continued to share moments of beauty amidst the pain—her daughters' laughter, Bruce's smiles, and the quiet grace of ordinary days. She reminded people that advocacy does not have to look like a protest or a speech. Sometimes, it is as simple as holding someone's hand, telling the truth, or choosing love over fear.

Her journey highlighted an important truth: visibility is powerful. When people see someone they admire facing hardship with authenticity, it shifts the conversation. Dementia, often spoken about in hushed tones or avoided altogether, was now being discussed openly in living rooms and classrooms. People were researching the signs, talking to doctors, checking in on their loved ones. This ripple effect was not accidental—it was the result of Emma's bravery.

In sharing her story, Emma also broke open the myth that caregiving is a solitary role. She highlighted the need for community, for shared knowledge, and for national conversations about elder care and medical support. She inspired other public figures to speak out about their experiences, helping to normalize the complexities of caregiving and illness in the public sphere.

Her influence extended to the media, where coverage of Bruce's condition began to reflect a deeper sense of empathy and responsibility. Instead of sensationalizing his decline, many outlets began focusing on the reality of dementia and the importance of early diagnosis. This shift was, in no small part, due to the tone Emma set—measured, informative, and rooted in love.

Emma also recognized the power of storytelling as advocacy. Through essays, interviews, and even informal conversations, she used narrative to build bridges. She told the story of a woman who never expected to become a caregiver, who wrestled with guilt, fatigue, and heartbreak, but who found strength in purpose. She told the story of a family reshaped by illness, and the love that held them together. These stories, grounded in truth, became tools for empathy.

Voicing the journey also meant inviting others to step into their own roles as advocates. Emma encouraged followers to share their stories, to volunteer, to donate, to reach out. She made it clear that advocacy is not reserved for celebrities or experts—it belongs to anyone willing to speak, to act, and to care. Her platform became a kind of gathering place for collective action, where people from all walks of life could come together with one shared goal: to create a world where no one faces dementia alone.

She continued to evolve her message, recognizing that awareness is just the beginning. Advocacy requires sustained effort, uncomfortable conversations, and systemic change. Emma began supporting legislative efforts around increased research funding for neurological diseases, and joined voices calling for national caregiver support initiatives. She worked to ensure that families like hers, navigating the storm of dementia, were not overlooked.

Through all of this, she stayed true to her values—compassion, authenticity, and love. Her advocacy was not born out of ambition, but out of necessity. And that, perhaps, is why it resonates so deeply. It comes from the place where the personal meets the political, where grief becomes a bridge to empathy, and where pain becomes the catalyst for change.

In raising her voice, Emma gave others the courage to raise theirs. And in doing so, she transformed a private heartbreak into a public mission. One that educates, inspires, and connects. One that insists on dignity for those living with dementia. One that honors the caregivers whose love is fierce and unrelenting. One that proves that when we use our platforms for good, we do more than speak—we move.

Emma Heming Willis did not choose this path. But in walking it with grace, she has become not just a voice, but a movement. A reminder that stories heal, that truth matters, and that the most powerful platform we have is the one we use to lift others up.

Chapter Seven

Hope in the Everyday: Finding Beauty, Humor, and Humanity in the Hardest Times

There is a certain kind of hope that is not loud. It does not shout from mountaintops or declare itself in grand speeches. It whispers in the quiet spaces of ordinary life. It waits patiently in the pause between heartbreaks. It appears in the warmth of a child's laughter, the comfort of a familiar song, or the simple act of making breakfast while the world feels like it is unraveling. This kind of hope is what Emma Heming Willis has come to know deeply. Not the abstract kind, but the living, breathing, ever-present form of hope that shows up when you least expect it—and precisely when you need it most.

When Bruce Willis was diagnosed with frontotemporal dementia, the world shifted beneath Emma's feet. Suddenly, everything became sharper and softer all at once. The stakes of each moment grew higher, and the beauty within those moments grew richer. It was as if time had taken on a new texture, one that required her to pay close attention to what once seemed routine. Life no longer moved in fast motion. It slowed, deepened, and invited her to look again—to see not only the sorrow, but the wonder that still lingered in every corner of her days.

At first, finding beauty in the midst of grief felt almost impossible. The initial wave of the diagnosis had left her breathless. She was managing medical appointments, caring for her daughters, learning the language of a disease that would slowly take pieces of her husband away. There were days when even breathing felt like a task. And yet, in the thick of it all, hope began to bloom—not in dramatic gestures, but in the smallest of details.

One morning, while preparing breakfast for her daughters, Emma watched as Bruce slowly entered the room. He smiled, a little slower than before, but with the same warmth that had once captivated audiences on screen. He kissed their girls on their heads, tousled their hair, and sat beside them. In that moment, nothing else mattered—not the disease, not the future, not the weight of what was coming. What mattered was the love at that table, the joy in their children's eyes, and the sense that, despite everything, life was still happening and it was still beautiful.

It was in moments like these that Emma discovered the resilience of the human spirit. She learned that humor and heartbreak often walk side by side. Sometimes Bruce would say something that made no logical sense, but the way he said it—his delivery, his expression, his timing—made the entire room burst into laughter. The disease was robbing him of certain faculties, yes, but it had not stolen his essence. His charm, his light, his connection to those he loved—those remained.

Laughter, Emma found, was not a betrayal of the pain, but a necessary companion to it. It kept them all human. It reminded them that while dementia could touch many things, it could not touch the core of who they were as a family. There was grace in the silliness, in the shared glances that communicated a kind of secret courage, in the inside jokes that only grew stronger as their world grew more tender.

Emma began to practice the art of noticing. She started to keep a gratitude journal, not because she wanted to mask her grief, but because she needed a way to ground herself. Some days, her entries were short: "The way Bruce smiled at me this morning," or "The sound of the girls singing in the bathroom." Other days, they were more detailed, reflections on the smell of coffee, the feel of sunlight on her face, the kindness of a stranger who recognized her but said nothing, offering only a smile. These small acts of awareness became lifelines.

Hope, she realized, was not something you stumbled upon. It was something you chose. Not always easily, and not always right away, but again and again, in the face of difficulty. It was in the decision to get up and make the bed. To go for a walk. To call a friend. To take a photo of Bruce when he was at ease. These choices, though mundane, were sacred. They were acts of resistance against despair.

Motherhood, too, offered a profound window into hope. Watching her daughters grow, laugh, and adapt to their father's changing condition filled Emma with awe. Children have a way of seeing what matters. They do not carry the same kind of fear about the future. Instead, they live in the now. They dance when there is music, they ask questions when they are curious, and they love without restraint. Emma watched her girls care for Bruce in ways that were pure and instinctive. They held his hand, made him drawings, sat beside him while watching movies. Their presence was a balm.

In their innocence, Emma found strength. They were not weighed down by the medical terms or the prognosis. They simply loved. They taught her that you do not have to understand everything to be fully present. That sometimes the best thing you can do for someone you love is just to be near them, to share space and time without needing to fix what is broken.

As Emma leaned deeper into these lessons, she also found healing in connection with others. Her decision to speak publicly about Bruce's condition created a ripple effect. Strangers reached out to share their own stories of caregiving, of grief, of finding light in the shadows. These connections reminded her that she was not alone. That others, too, were living through unimaginable circumstances and still finding reasons to laugh, to dance, to hope.

She formed friendships with other caregivers— some famous, some not—who understood what it meant to live in the tension between acceptance and advocacy. They traded tips, stories, encouragement. They spoke of sleepless nights and miraculous mornings. Of the guilt that sometimes clings to caregivers like a second skin. And of the sacred moments that catch you off guard and fill your chest with light.

Emma began to see her life as a tapestry. Not seamless or perfect, but rich with texture and meaning. The hard days were still hard. There were still moments of exhaustion, of frustration, of grief so deep it stole the air from her lungs. But there were also moments of grace—when Bruce said something unexpectedly tender, when the girls wrapped their arms around her at just the right time, when a nurse offered compassion, or a friend showed up without being asked.

The beauty, she discovered, was not in the absence of pain, but in the presence of love despite the pain. In the way her family kept showing up for one another. In the quiet rhythm of daily rituals—brushing Bruce's hair, walking him through the garden, reading aloud from a favorite book. These acts became ceremonies of hope, reminders that even as the disease progressed, life continued to offer opportunities for connection and meaning.

Art also became a refuge. Music, photography, storytelling—these outlets allowed Emma and her family to express what words sometimes could not. Music, in particular, had a unique power. There were days when Bruce would respond to songs in ways he no longer responded to speech. A melody could stir a memory, a smile, a subtle movement of his hand. Emma began to curate playlists that brought comfort and familiarity. The girls danced. Bruce watched with a twinkle in his eye. These were the moments that reminded her that joy was still possible.

Even in the chaos of caregiving, Emma learned to find rhythm. She embraced slowness, let go of perfection, and began to value presence over productivity. A successful day was no longer measured by tasks completed, but by the depth of connection shared. Had she held Bruce's hand? Had she made the girls laugh? Had she taken a moment to breathe, to be, to honor herself?

She spoke more openly about mental health, about the emotional toll of caregiving and the importance of seeking help. Hope, she believed, required honesty. It required naming the hard things, so that they would not consume you. Therapy, rest, asking for support—these became part of her healing. She began to dismantle the myth that strength meant doing it all alone. Real strength, she found, was in letting others in.

In the end, it was not the grand gestures that sustained her, but the everyday acts of love. The meals shared, the hands held, the stories told. The decision, again and again, to choose grace over bitterness. To believe that there is beauty in the broken places. To trust that even in the shadow of illness, the light still finds its way through.

Emma's journey with Bruce, with their girls, with this new chapter of life, has not been one of easy answers. But it has been one of deep truth. Of discovering that hope is not the absence of struggle, but the resolve to face it with open eyes and an open heart. That beauty can live inside pain. That humor can break through silence. That love, in all its forms, endures.

Hope in the everyday is not flashy or loud. It is tender. It is steady. It is the hand on your back when you feel like falling, the voice that says you are not alone, the breath you take when the world feels like too much. It is the truth that even now, even here, life is worth loving. And that is what Emma holds onto. Not because it is easy, but because it is real.

Conclusion
Still With Love: The Ongoing Story of Compassion, Connection, and Courage

There are stories that do not end with a final sentence, a last scene, or a moment of resolution. There are stories that live on through breath, memory, and presence— through the heartbeat of a family still choosing each other every day. Emma Heming Willis has come to understand that hers is such a story. One without a neat conclusion, one that defies tidy bows or finished chapters. A story where love continues even in uncertainty, where courage takes the shape of showing up, and where connection is not a luxury but a necessity.

When the diagnosis of frontotemporal dementia entered Emma and Bruce's life, it did not arrive quietly. It carved into their world a new and unfamiliar landscape—one where grief lived beside joy, and fear walked hand in hand with love. It stripped away illusions, demanded honesty, and forced a reimagining of what it means to be a family, a partner, a caregiver, and most importantly, a human being. But in this shifting terrain, Emma found something enduring. Not the kind of strength forged in denial, but a deeper kind of bravery born from compassion, connection, and radical presence.

Compassion became her compass. Not just for Bruce, but for herself. At the beginning, Emma believed she needed to carry everything alone. There was a silent expectation she placed on herself to be perfect, to protect her children, to maintain appearances, to never let the world see her crack. But the reality of caregiving refused to be wrapped in perfection. There were sleepless nights, tears shed in laundry rooms, moments of frustration that brought her to her knees. And still, there was love. Love in the way she adjusted Bruce's collar before an interview. Love in the way she smiled through exhaustion so her daughters would feel safe. Love in the way she allowed herself, finally, to be vulnerable.

True compassion, she learned, begins when we allow ourselves to feel—to grieve, to rage, to rest. It is the choice to soften rather than harden, to let in support rather than wall it off.

Compassion says it is okay to not be okay. It says you are worthy of care even as you give it to others. Emma learned to forgive herself for the days she felt overwhelmed, to ask for help when she needed it, and to receive love without guilt.

Connection became her lifeline. The more she opened her heart publicly, the more hands reached out in response. Caregivers from across the world messaged her stories that mirrored her own—quiet warriors walking through similar fires. They shared what it meant to love someone who was changing, to carry the weight of memory alone, to choose presence in the face of loss. Emma no longer felt isolated. She felt part of a sacred, unseen community—a sisterhood of strength, tenderness, and resilience.

She nurtured relationships within her own home with the same intentionality. Her daughters were growing, absorbing everything, watching how she responded to pain. She wanted to show them not just survival, but the beauty of transformation. She involved them in Bruce's care, allowing them to experience both the challenge and the joy of showing up for someone they love. Together, they sang, played, laughed, and held space for one another's tears. Emma understood that this was not just about caregiving. It was about legacy. About raising daughters who would know what love looks like when it is tested, what strength sounds like when it whispers, and what kindness feels like in the middle of difficulty.

Courage became her anthem. Not the loud, roaring courage of battlefields, but the quiet kind that shows up in the everyday. The courage to stay when things are hard. To speak truthfully about grief and mental health. To advocate publicly not just for Bruce, but for others like him, for the caregivers whose voices are often silenced, for the families who are walking similar paths and do not yet know they are not alone. Courage, Emma discovered, is built in the quiet rituals—the brushing of teeth, the morning tea, the holding of hands. It is built in choosing tenderness over withdrawal, laughter over bitterness, hope over resignation.

She continued to use her platform not to paint a portrait of perfect caregiving, but to reflect the realness of it. She shared the beautiful moments—the milestones, the smiles, the victories of love—and she shared the hard ones too. The confusion, the exhaustion, the longing for the way things used to be. She dismantled the myth that caregiving is only noble. It is also deeply human. Messy. Complicated. Sacred.

Still, love endured. That was the truth she returned to again and again. Love is not undone by illness. It does not wither when memory fades. It may change its shape, its language, its expression, but it remains. Bruce, even in his evolving state, still offered moments of connection. A glance. A smile. A soft word. And Emma received these with open arms, collecting them like treasures. They were reminders that he was still with her—not in the same way as before, but in a way that was no less meaningful.

This journey also transformed Emma's sense of purpose. She had once walked the runways of Paris and New York. She had stood in front of cameras, posed for covers, attended glamorous events. But now, her spotlight had shifted. She stood as a voice for those who needed visibility. For caregivers. For women learning to balance motherhood with medical caregiving. For families navigating brain disorders with too few resources. For anyone who has had to choose love in the presence of loss.

She leaned into education and advocacy with grace. She used her influence to raise awareness about frontotemporal dementia, to push for funding, to humanize the diagnosis. She partnered with experts, collaborated with nonprofits, and turned her pain into purpose. But even more, she remained grounded in what mattered most: home, love, and being present.

In the simplest of terms, Emma made a choice. To live fully. Not waiting for life to feel easy or perfect again. But embracing it as it is—raw, complicated, and breathtakingly real. She chose to find beauty in unexpected places. In her daughters' laughter, in the sunlight falling across Bruce's face, in the kindness of strangers, in the wisdom that only suffering can teach. She chose to love Bruce not for who he was in the past, but for who he continued to be—here and now.

Their love story had taken a new form. It was not the Hollywood romance of red carpets and headlines. It was something richer. A story of commitment, sacrifice, devotion, and depth. A love that bore the weight of a diagnosis and still stood tall. A love that adapted, endured, and evolved.

As Emma looks forward, she does not pretend to know what the future holds. The road ahead is still uncertain. There will be more hard days. More letting go. More moments when the ache feels unbearable. But there will also be beauty. There will be birthdays, family dinners, quiet walks, unexpected joy. There will be new memories made in the context of change. And most importantly, there will still be love.

This is the story that continues. One of a woman who did not choose her circumstances, but who chose how to meet them. With courage. With compassion. With connection. Emma's life is not defined by tragedy. It is defined by the grace with which she responds to it. By the way she honors her husband. By the way she mothers her daughters. By the way she opens her life to others so they might find light in the dark.

Still with love. That is the heartbeat of this journey. A declaration that says, even now, even here, even in the silence of forgetting and the quiet of change, love remains. It is the steady hand, the patient presence, the soft-spoken truth. It is what carries them forward.

For Emma Heming Willis, caregiving is no longer just a role. It is a calling. A mission. A testimony. She is no longer only a wife, a mother, a public figure. She is a storyteller of the human condition. A witness to love that survives. And an example of how, even when everything shifts, we can still live beautifully.

The journey continues. But now it is bathed in deeper light, grounded in fuller truth, and held together by a kind of love that does not end.

Still with love. Always with love.

Made in the USA
Middletown, DE
27 August 2025

13106046R00060